Mediterranean Diet Recipes

A Simplified Guide To To Lose Weight, Feel Great, And Improve Your Overall Health By Following The Mediterranean Diet For Weight Loss

By

Grace Morelli

Table Of Contents

Introduction

Thank you very much for purchasing this book. The Mediterranean diet includes foods that can help reduce heart attack and stroke and also decrease risk factors, including obesity, high cholesterol, high blood pressure, and diabetes. The Mediterranean has a high intake of virgin olive oil which allows the body to remove a lot of cholesterol from the blood vessels and keep the arteries open. Eating with family and friends, drinking a bottle of red wine and becoming socially involved are also vital aspects of the Mediterranean lifestyle.

Enjoy your meal.

Mediterranean Smoothies Recipes

Kale-Pineapple Smoothie

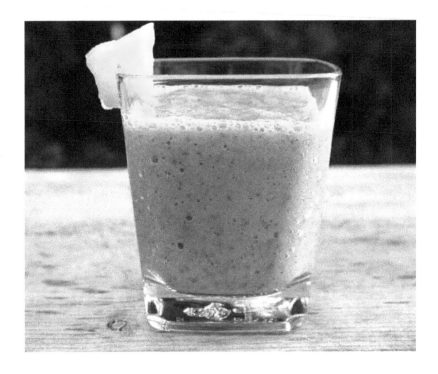

(Prep time: 10 minutes | Blend time: 2 minutes |Servings: 1)

Nutrition: 107 Cal | 5.9 g Fat |11 g Carbs |5 g Protein

Ingredients

- 1 cucumber

- Honey: 1 tbsp.

- Fresh mint, as required

- Baby kale: ¼ pound

- Coconut milk: 1 cup

- Pineapple pieces: 1½ cups

Instructions

- Add all ingredients to the blender. Pulse on high until smooth and creamy.

- Serve right away.

Pineapple Green Smoothie

(Prep time: 10 minutes | Blend time: 2 minutes |Servings: 1)

Nutrition: 103 Cal | 8.3 g Fat |11.2 g Carbs | 6 g Protein

Ingredients

- Almond milk: half cup, chilled & unsweetened

- Baby spinach: 1 cup

- Greek yogurt: 1/3 cup, nonfat plain

- Pineapple chunks: half cup, frozen

- Banana: 1 cup, sliced

- Maple syrup: 1 tsp.

- Chia seeds: 1 tbsp.

Instructions

- Add all ingredients to the blender. Pulse on high until smooth and creamy.

- Serve right away.

Antioxidant Power Smoothie

(Prep time: 10 minutes | Blend time: 2 minutes |Servings: 1)

Nutrition: 99 Cal | 3 g Fat |13 g Carbs |8 g Protein

Ingredients

- Honey: 1 tbsp.

- Fresh blueberries: 1 cup

- Blueberry yogurt: ¾ cup

- Fresh blackberries: 1 cup

- Pomegranate juice: half cup

Instructions

- Add all ingredients to the blender. Pulse on high until smooth and creamy.

- Serve right away.

Mediterranean Breakfast Recipes

Easy Breakfast Stuffed Peppers

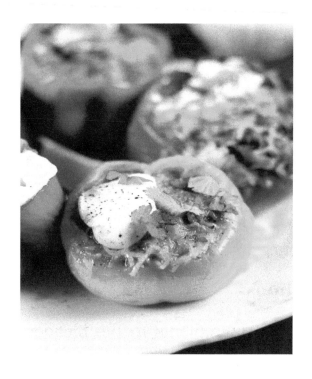

(Prep time: 10 minutes | Cook time: 30 minutes |Servings: 5-6)

Nutrition: 224 Cal 20 g Fat |15.9 g Carbs |17 g Protein

Ingredients

- Olive oil, as needed

- 3 bell peppers, halved lengthwise and emptied

- Water, as needed

- Chopped yellow onion: 1 cup

- Peeled potatoes: 10-12 oz., diced

- 3 minced garlic cloves

- Mushrooms: 6 oz., chopped

- Salt & black pepper, to taste

- Chopped cherry tomatoes: half cup

- Aleppo pepper: ¾ tsp.

- Coriander: ¾ tsp.

- 6 eggs

- Organic cumin: ¾ tsp.

- Turmeric: half tsp.

- Chopped fresh parsley, packed: half cup

Instructions

- Let the oven preheat to 350 F.

- Place the half peppers in the baking dish. Add water (1 cup) in the baking dish, cover with aluminum foil and bake for 10-15 minutes.

- Place a cast-iron skillet on high flame, add mushrooms, salt and cook until browned. Take them out on a plate.

- Add olive oil to the skillet (2 tbsp.) add potatoes and onion in hot oil.

- Season with salt, pepper and other spices. Cook for five minutes and add garlic cook for 5-7 minutes on medium flame until potatoes become tender.

- Add mushrooms, parsley and tomatoes. Mix well and turn off the heat.

- Take peppers out from the oven, discard the water and stuff the mixture into the peppers, 3/4 of the way. Put one egg on top of the stuffing.

- Cover with foil and bake for 18-20 minutes.

- Serve right away.

Easy Muesli

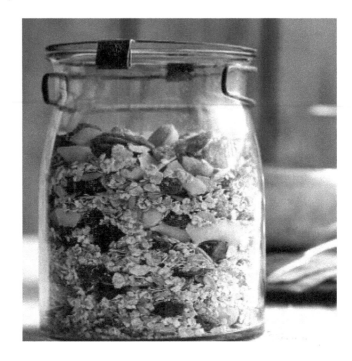

(Prep time: 10 minutes | Cook time: 20 minutes |Servings: 8)

Nutrition: 275 Cal | 13.0 g Fat |36.4 g Carbs |8.5 g Protein

Ingredients

- Wheat bran: half cup

- Kosher salt: half tsp.

- Coconut flakes, unsweetened: half cup

- Ground cinnamon: half tsp.

- Dried cherries: 1/4 cup

- Rolled oats: 3 1/2 cups

- Sliced almonds: half cup

- Raw pepitas: 1/4 cup

- Raw pecans: 1/4 cup, roughly chopped

- Dried apricots: 1/4 cup, coarsely chopped

Instructions

- Let the oven preheat to 350 F with 2 racks.

- Place wheat bran, salt, cinnamon and oats on a baking sheet and toss well, make into one even layer.

- In another baking sheet, add pepitas, almonds, and pecans. Toss and make into an even layer. Roast for 10-12 minutes by placing oats on the top rack and the nuts on the lower rack.

- Take the nuts' baking sheet out and let it cool.

- Sprinkle coconuts over oats, and bake again for five minutes. Take out and let it cool for ten minutes.

- In large bowls, add all contents of both baking sheets.

- Add cherries and apricot; toss well.

- Store in an airtight jar and use for 1 month.

Snow Pea & Ricotta Toasts

(Prep time: 10 minutes | Cook time: 0 minutes |Servings: 4)

Nutrition: 131 Cal | 5.5 g Fat |17 g Carbs |8.5 g Protein

Ingredients

- Snow peas: 4 oz.

- Salt: half tsp.

- White wine vinegar: 1 tbsp.

- Olive oil: 1 tbsp.

- Ricotta: 4 oz.

- Prepared horseradish: 2 tsp.

- Honey: half tsp.

- 4 slices of toasted bread

Instructions

- Cut peas in ¼ inch thick crosswise. In a bowl, whisk the rest of the ingredients with snow peas except for bread and ricotta.

- On each toast slice, spread one oz. of ricotta and serve with snow peas mixture on top.

White Beans with Greens & Poached Egg

(Prep time: 10 minutes | Cook time: 0 minutes |Servings: 4)

Nutrition: 301 Cal | 15.5 g Fat |26.5 g Carbs |15 g Protein

Ingredients

- Za'atar: 2 tsp.

- 3 tablespoons olive oil

- 4 eggs, poached

- 2 minced garlic cloves

- Kosher salt: 1 tsp.

- Swiss chard: ~10 oz., stems removed & leaves sliced

- 1 can of (15-oz.) cannellini beans, rinsed

- Red pepper flakes: 1/4 tsp.

- Lemon juice: 1 tbsp.

Instructions

- In a pan, add oil (2 tbsp.) on medium flame until hot.

- Add beans and cook for 2-4 minutes.

- Add za'atar (1 tsp.) and salt (half tsp.), mix well.

- Cook for 3-5 minutes, until beans are golden brown, take them out on a plate.

- Add oil (1 tbsp.) to the pan, add chard and season with the rest of the za'atar, salt, cook for 3-5 minutes.

- Turn off the heat and add lemon juice and toss well.

- In four bowls, add beans and place a poached egg on top with red pepper flakes. Serve right away.

Zucchini with Eggs

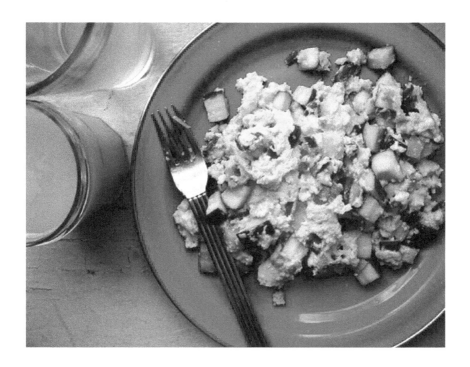

(Prep time: 10 minutes | Cook time: 5-7 minutes |Servings: 2)

Nutrition: 111 Cal | 12 g Fat |21 g Carbs |16 g Protein

Ingredients

- Salt & black pepper, to taste

- Olive oil: 1 ½ tbsp.

- Water: 1 tsp.

- 2 zucchinis, sliced into large chunks

- 2 eggs

Instructions

- In a skillet, add oil and sauté zucchini for ten minutes until tender. Season with salt and black pepper.

- Whisk eggs in a bowl with water. Pour eggs over zucchini, cook until eggs are scrambled and sprinkle salt and pepper on top.

- Serve right away.

Mediterranean Poultry Recipes

Greek Stuffed Chicken

(Prep time: 15 minutes| Cook time: 35 minutes |Servings: 4)

Nutrition: 387 Cal | 21 g Fat |17 g Carbs |34 g Protein

Ingredients

- Olive oil: 3 tbsp.

- 4 chicken breasts, skinless & boneless

- Lemon juice: 1 tbsp.

- Chopped parsley: 1 tbsp.

- Chopped dill: 1 tbsp.

- 2 minced garlic cloves

- 2 lemons, half-moons

- 1 zucchini, half-moons

- Shredded mozzarella: 1 cup

- 2 tomatoes, half-moons

- Salt & black pepper, to taste

- Half red onion, half-moons

- Crumbled feta: 1 cup

Instructions

- Let the oven preheat to 400 F.

- Make five cuts in every chicken breast, do not slice all the way through.

- In a bowl, add all ingredients except for all vegetables and cheeses. Mix and pour over chicken breast and season with salt and pepper.

- Stuff the chicken with all half-moons, and sprinkle both kinds of cheese on top.

- Bake on a baking sheet for 25 minutes.

- Serve right away.

Baked Chicken Thighs

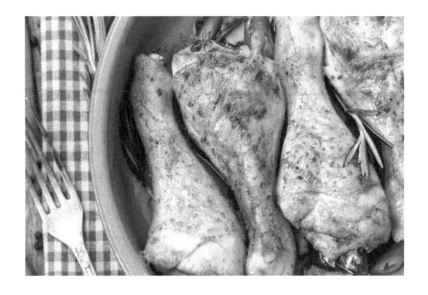

(Prep time: 10 minutes| Cook time: 40 minutes |Servings: 8)

Nutrition: 313 Cal | 28 g Fat |9 g Carbs |20 g Protein

Ingredients

- 3 yellow onions, sliced thin

- 8 chicken thighs, with skin & bone

- 1 tomato, sliced

- Kosher Salt, to taste

For the chicken rub

- Smoked paprika: 1 tsp.

- Olive oil: ⅓ cup

- 1 lemon's juice

- Tomato paste: 5 tbsp.

- Black pepper: 1 tsp.

- Dry oregano: 1 tsp.

- 4 minced garlic cloves

- Cumin: 1 tsp.

Instructions

- Let the oven preheat to 425 F.

- With the salt season, the chicken thighs generously.

- In a bowl, add all the rub ingredients and mix well.

- Coat the chicken well in this rub mixture and under the skin too.

- Oil spray a 9 by 13" of the baking tray, add onions on the bottom.

- Place chicken on top, and add water (1/4 cup) on the sides.

- Bake for 40 minutes, broil for few minutes if needed. Serve right away.

Mediterranean Chicken Skillet

(Prep time: 20 minutes| Cook time: 40 minutes |Servings: 8)

Nutrition: 232 Cal | 8 g Fat |5 g Carbs |33 g Protein

Ingredients

- Coriander: half tsp.

- Chicken breasts: 2 lb., boneless skinless

- Onion powder: 1 tsp.

- Crushed red pepper, to taste

- 2 sliced garlic cloves

- Paprika: half tsp.

- Olive oil: 2 tbsp.

- Yellow onion: 1 cup, chopped

- Black olives: ¼ cup, sliced

- Salt & black pepper, to taste

- Diced tomatoes: 1 ½ cups

- Feta cheese: 2 tbsp.

Instructions

- Let the oven preheat to 400 F.

- In a bowl, add all spices, mix and add chicken. Coat it well.

- In a skillet, brown the chicken on medium flame. Take out on a plate.

- Add onions, cook for 3 to 5 minutes.

- Add garlic, cook for half a minute, then add tomatoes. Mix well.

- Place chicken back in the pan. Bake for 20 minutes in the oven until the internal temperature of the chicken reaches 165 F.

- Serve with cheese and olives on top.

Slow-Cooked Moroccan Chicken

(Prep time: 20 minutes| Cook time: 6 hours |Servings: 4)

Nutrition: 435 Cal | 9 g Fat |32 g Carbs |42 g Protein

Ingredients

- 4 carrots, sliced

- (3-4 pounds) fryer chicken cut up without skin

- Salt: half tsp.

- All-purpose flour: 2 tbsp.

- Tomato paste: 1/4 cup

- Chopped dried apricots: half cup

- Raisins: half cup

- Onions, sliced in half moons

- 1 can of (~15 oz.) Chicken broth

- Ground cumin: 1 ½ tsp.

- Lemon juice: 2 tbsp.

- Pepper: 3/4 tsp.

- Minced garlic cloves

- Ground ginger: 1 ½ tsp.

- Ground cinnamon: 1 tsp.

Instructions

- Season the chicken with salt.

- In a slow cooker (5 qt.), add onion, carrots and seasoned chicken.

- Add raisins, apricots to the cooker.

- In a bowl, add the rest of the ingredients, mix well and pour into the slow cooker.

- Cook on low for 6 to 7 hours. Serve with couscous.

Turkey Kibbeh

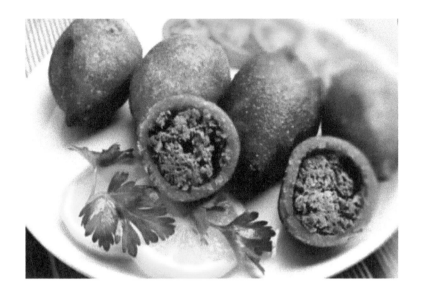

(Prep time: 10 minutes| Cook time: 1 hour|Servings: 6)

Nutrition: 415 Cal | 11 g Fat |38 g Carbs |28 g Protein

Ingredients

- Olive oil: 1 tbsp.

- Toasted pine nuts: 1/4 cup

- Bulgur: half cup

- Ground cumin: 1 ½ tsp.

- Lean ground turkey: 1 ½ pound

- Kosher salt: 1 ½ tsp.

- Zucchini, shredded

- 1 onion, diced

- Cayenne pepper: ¼ tsp.

- Dried marjoram: 2 tsp.

- Ground allspice: half tsp.

Yogurt sauce

- Tomato, diced

- Plain yogurt: 1 cup

- Black pepper, to taste

- Half cucumber, diced without seeds

Instructions

- Let the oven preheat to 450 F, and oil spray an 8" baking dish (square).

- Put bulgur in hot water and cover the pan.

- In a skillet, add oil and sauté onion for 4 minutes. Turn off the heat and add pine nuts.

- Discard the liquid from the bulgur, and take it out in a bowl.

- Add the rest of the ingredients to the bowl. Mix gently.

- Put half of the mixture in the baking dish and add onions on top in one layer.

- Add the rest of the meat mixture on top. Cover with aluminum foil.

- Bake for half an hour. Take the foil off and bake for 10-15 minutes more until the meat's internal temperature reaches 165 F.

- In a bowl, add all ingredients of yogurt sauce mix and serve with kibbeh.

Mediterranean Appetizers & Sides Recipes

All-Green Crudités Basket

(Prep time: 9 minutes | Cook time: 1 minutes |Servings: 8)

Nutrition: 57 Cal | 1 g Fat | 12 g Carbs |5 g Protein

Ingredients

- String beans: 8 oz., trimmed

- Celery: 1 bunch, cut into sticks

- Broccoli: 1 head, broken into florets

- 3 heads large leaves endive, cut in half lengthwise

- Fennel: 1 bulb, cut into thin vertical slices

- Cucumber, cut into matchsticks

- 1 green pepper, sliced with seeds

Instructions

- Boil water in a large pot, and fill one pot with ice water.

- Add the broccoli, beans into boiling water for 1 minute. Then transfer to ice water.

- Take out and dry.

- In a basket, place all vegetables in small clusters and serve with dipping.

Falafel Smash

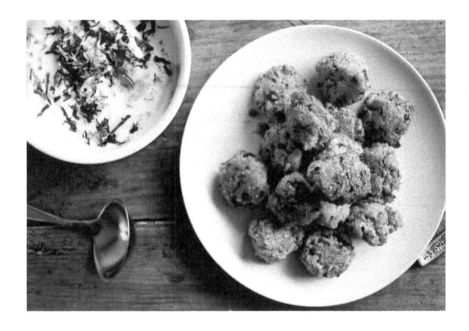

(Prep time: 10 minutes | Cook time: 5 minutes |Servings: 3-4)

Nutrition: 278 Cal | 7 g Fat | 28 g Carbs |5 g Protein

Ingredients

- Salt: ¼ tsp.

- Olive oil: 1 tbsp.

- Ground cumin: 1 tsp.

- Ground coriander: 1 tsp.

- Non-dairy yogurt: 1/4 cup

- Red pepper flakes: ¼ tsp.

- Cooked chickpeas: 1 1/2 cups

- Half lemon's juice

- 4 to 6 pita breads

- Arugula: 1 cup

- Pickled red onion: few slices

Cilantro Sauce

- 1 Minced garlic clove

- Salt, to taste

- Toasted sesame seeds: 2 tbsp.

- Cilantro: 2 cups chopped w/stems

- Olive oil: 1/4 cup

Instructions

- In a bowl, mash the cooked chickpeas lightly.

- Add spices, oil and lemon juice to the chickpeas and mix.

- In a bowl, add the ingredients of the sauce, mix well.

- On the bread, add yogurt, arugula, then chickpeas and sauce. Top with picked slices and serve

Crab Phyllo Cups

(Prep time: 10 minutes | Cook time: 0 minutes |Servings: 14)

Nutrition: 34 Cal | 2 g Fat | 3 g Carbs |1 g Protein

Ingredients

- Lump crabmeat: 3/4 cup, drained

- Vegetable cream cheese (spreadable): half cup

- Chili sauce: 5 tbsp.

- Seafood seasoning: half tsp.

- 2 packs of (1.9 oz. each) miniature tart phyllo shells

Instructions

- In a bowl, mix cream cheese with seasoning, fold in crab.

- In each tart shell, add 2 tsp. of cream cheese mix, add chili sauce on top and serve

Baked Zucchini with Parmesan & Thyme

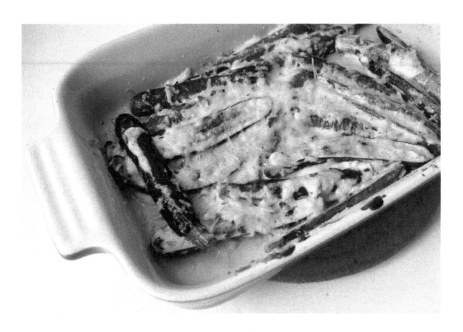

(Prep time: 10 minutes | Cook time: 18 minutes |Servings: 5)

Nutrition: 66 Cal | 3.3 g Fat |4.8 g Carbs |4.8 g Protein

Ingredients

- 3-4 zucchini, cut length-wise into sticks

- Olive oil

Parmesan & Thyme Topping

- Dried oregano: 1 tsp.

- Grated parmesan cheese: half cup

- Kosher salt, a pinch

- Black pepper: half tsp.

- Fresh thyme leaves: 2 tsp.

- Sweet paprika: half tsp.

Instructions

- Let the oven preheat to 350 f.

- In a bowl, mix spices, parmesan and thyme.

- Place a wire rack on a baking sheet and oil spray with olive oil.

- Place the zucchini, skin side down on the rack and brush with oil.

- Sprinkle with parmesan topping.

- Bake for 15-20 minutes, broil for 2-3 minutes.

- Serve right away.

Mediterranean Fish & Seafood Recipes

Harissa Stew with Eggplant & Millet

(Prep time: 35 minutes | Cook time: 10 minutes |Servings: 1)

Nutrition: 600 Cal | 15 g Fat | 88 g Carbs 20 g Protein

Ingredients

- Millet: 1 cup

- Ghee: 2 tbsp.

- 1 Can of (14 oz.) Puréed tomatoes

- Kosher salt, to taste

- Black pepper

- 1 onion, chopped

- Harissa paste: 2 tbsp.

- 1 Japanese eggplant

- 3 Minced garlic cloves

- 1 can of (14 oz.) chickpeas, drained

Instructions

- In a pan, add water (2 cups), salt and millet. Cook covered for 25 minutes. Fluff with a fork and let it cool.

- In a skillet, add ghee (1 tbsp.), add eggplant and season with salt and pepper; cook for ten minutes, add more ghee if necessary.

- Take out on a plate.

- Sauté onion for 8-10 minutes.

- Add garlic, cook for 2 minutes. Add salt, pepper, tomato, harissa and chickpeas. Mix and add eggplant back in the pan.

- Turn the heat low and let it simmer for 10-15 minutes.

- On top of millet, serve the stew.

Salmon Bowl with Tahini

(Prep time: 10 minutes | Cook time: 30 minutes |Servings: 1)

Nutrition: 1732 Cal | 137 g Fat | 81 g Carbs | 59 g Protein

Ingredients

- Tahini: 2 tbsp.

- Turmeric: half tsp.

- Olive oil: 6 tbsp.

- Zest & juice of 1 lemon

- Salt & black pepper, to taste

- Salmon: 6 oz.

- Farro: ¼ cup

- Coriander: half tsp.

- Black beans: half cup, cooked

- Garlic powder: ¼ tsp.

- Cumin: half tsp.

- Smoked paprika: 1 ½ tsp.

- ¼ Fresno Chile, sliced thin

- 4 lettuce leaves

Instructions

- In a bowl, whisk garlic powder, tahini, juice, zest and turmeric (1/4 tsp.).

- Mix and add olive oil (3 tbsp.) while keep whisking. Whisk until emulsified.

- Add salt and pepper.

- Cook farro in water (1 cup) for 20-25 minutes.

- In a bowl, toss beans with olive oil (1 tbsp.) and cumin.

- Season the fish with the rest of the ingredients except for lettuce leaves, Chile.

- Cook salmon in pan for five minutes, till it cooks.

- In the serving bowl, add lettuce leaves, farro, salmon and top with black beans and chile.

Greek Roasted Fish with Vegetables

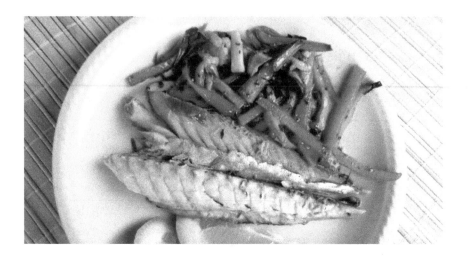

(Prep time: 35 minutes | Cook time: 20 minutes |Servings: 4)

Nutrition: 422 Cal | 18.6 g Fat | 31.5 g Carbs | 32.9 g Protein

Ingredients

• Fingerling potatoes: 1 pound, cut in half vertically

• Olive oil: 2 tbsp.

• 2 sweet peppers, cut into rounds

- 5 minced garlic cloves

- Black pepper: half tsp.

- 4 skinless salmon fillets

- Sea salt: half tsp.

- Kalamata olives: ¼ cup, halved

- Cherry tomatoes: 2 cups

- Fresh oregano: ¼ cup

- Chopped fresh parsley: 1 ½ cups

- 1 Lemon

Instructions

- Let the oven preheat to 425 F.

- In a bowl, add potatoes, and toss with salt, pepper, olive oil (1 tbsp.), and garlic.

- Place in a 15 by 10" baking pan, roast, covered for half an hour.

- In a bowl, add sweet peppers, salt, pepper, oregano, tomatoes, olives, parsley, and olive oil (1 tbsp.), toss.

- Season the fish with salt and pepper.

- On the baking pan, on top of potatoes, add sweet peppers and salmon.

- Roast for ten minutes, uncovered.

- Serve with lemon juice on top.

Salmon Souvlaki Bowls

(Prep time: 15 minutes | Cook time: 15 minutes |Servings: 4)

Nutrition: 422 Cal | 18.6 g Fat | 31.5 g Carbs | 32.9 g Protein

Ingredients

- Fresh salmon: 1 pound, cut into four pieces

- Olive oil: 3 tbsp.

- Lemon juice: 6 tbsp.

- 2 minced garlic cloves

- Balsamic vinegar: 2 tbsp.

- Smoked paprika: 1 tbsp.

- Salt: half tsp.

- Fresh dill: 1 tbsp.

- Pepper: 1 tsp.

- Fresh oregano: 1 tbsp.

Bowls

- Cherry tomatoes: 1 cup, halved

- 2 red peppers, cut into fours

- Kalamata olives: half cup

- Zucchini, cut into rounds

- Feta cheese crumbled: ¾ cup

- Dry farro: 1 cup

- Olive oil: 2 tbsp.

- 2 cucumbers, sliced thin

- 1 Lemon's juice

Instructions

- In a bowl, add all ingredients except for salmon mix and add salmon. Toss to coat.

- Let it marinate for 10 to 15 minutes.

- Cook farro, as per package instructions.

- In a bowl, add vegetables, and toss with olive oil, pepper and salt.

- Cook salmon on a grill pan for 3 minutes on one side. When flip, add the vegetables.

- Grill the vegetables.

- To serve, in serving bowls, add the farro and top with fish and grilled vegetables.

Mediterranean Meatless & Vegetarian Recipes

Vegan Moussaka

(Prep time: 30 minutes | Cook time: 30 minutes |Servings: 6)

Nutrition: 341 Cal | 17 g Fat |36 g Carbs | 36 g Protein

Ingredients

Tomato Sauce

- Tomato paste: 1 tbsp.

- Maple syrup: 1 tsp.

- 1 Can of (28 oz.) Plum tomatoes

- Cinnamon: 1/8 tsp.

- 2 Onions, chopped

- 2 Minced garlic cloves

- Cayenne pepper, a pinch

- Smoked tofu: 12 oz., firm

- Salt: half tsp.

- Black pepper: 1/8 tsp.

Eggplants

- 3 eggplants, medium-sized

- Olive oil: 1 tbsp.

Bechamel Sauce

- Salt: half tsp.

- Unsweetened almond milk: 2 ½ cups

- Potato starch: 2 tbsp.

- Ground nutmeg: 1/8 tsp.

- Nutritional yeast: 2 tbsp.

Instructions

• In a bowl, add the canned tomato juice, and dice the tomatoes.

• In a skillet, add the chopped tomatoes with juices on medium flame. Cook for ten minutes until it slightly thickens.

• Add cinnamon, tomato paste, pepper, maple syrup, and salt; cook for 2 minutes. Turn off the heat.

• Slice eggplants into 1" thick slices, brush both sides with olive oil, and sprinkle salt on them.

• In a skillet, fry the eggplants on both sides on medium flame. Take out on a plate.

• In the same pan, saute onion and garlic for 7 minutes, add tofu, and scramble.

• Cook for five minutes. Add tomato sauce and mix well. Turn off the heat.

• In a pan, add almond milk and the rest of the bechamel sauce's ingredients.

- Whisk well on medium flame and cook for 5 to 10 minutes until it thickens. Turn off the heat.

- Let the oven preheat to 400 F.

- In an oil sprayed baking dish, layer the eggplants, add tofu mixture on top, add the second layer of eggplant. Pour béchamel and spread.

- Bake for 25 to 30 minutes, add fresh herbs on top, and serve.

Greek Quesadillas

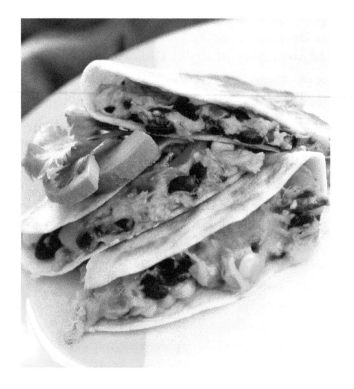

(Prep time: 20 minutes | Cook time: 10 minutes |Servings: 8)

Nutrition: 348 Cal | 18 g Fat |32 g Carbs | 14.4 g Protein

Ingredients

- 8 flour tortillas, 8"

- Mozzarella cheese: 1 cup, shredded

- Chopped spinach: 10 oz.

- Tzatziki sauce, as needed

- Kalamata olives: half cup, chopped

- Sun-dried tomatoes: half cup, in olive oil, chopped & drained

- Crumbled feta cheese: 1 cup

- Fresh dill: 1 tbsp.

Instructions

- Let the oven preheat to 400 F

- On the tortilla, spread the spinach, olives, tomatoes, cheese and place another tortilla on top.

- Make four quesadillas.

- Place these on a parchment-lined baking sheet, bake for 8 to 10 minutes.

- Serve with tzatziki sauce.

Vegetable Lentil Soup

(Prep time: 20 minutes | Cook time: 40 minutes |Servings: 8)

Nutrition: 284 Cal | 12 g Fat |18 g Carbs | 14.4 g Protein

Ingredients

- Olive oil: 2 tbsp.

- 2 cans of (15 oz.) Diced tomatoes, fire-roasted

- 2 large peeled carrots, chopped

- 5 minced garlic cloves

- 1 Onion, chopped

- Cumin: 2 tsp.

- Vegetable stock: 4 cups

- Dried thyme: half tsp.

- Red pepper flakes: half tsp.

- 1 can of (15 oz.) Chickpeas, rinsed

- Kale: 2 cups, chopped without ribs

- Pepper: 1 tsp.

- Water: 3 cups

- Green lentils: 1 cup

- Salt:1 tsp.

Instructions

- In a pot, add oil on medium flame. Saute onion, carrots until translucent and tender.

- Add thyme, garlic, and cumin. Cook for few minutes, add chickpeas and roasted tomatoes.

- Add vegetable stock, lentils, and water. Add pepper flakes, pepper, and salt.

- Let it come to a boil, turn the heat low and simmer for half an hour.

- Puree the soup with a stick blender to the consistency you like.

- Add kale, warm it through and serve.

Garlicky Swiss Chard & Chickpeas

(Prep time: 20 minutes | Cook time: 10 minutes |Servings: 2)

Nutrition: 498 Cal | 28 g Fat |43.7 g Carbs |15.8 g Protein

Ingredients

- Olive oil: 1 tbsp.

- Vegetable broth: 2 cups

- 1 Can of (15.5 oz.) Garbanzo beans, rinsed

- 2 Shallots, chopped

- 6 minced garlic cloves

- Swiss chard: 2 bunches, leaves roughly chopped

- Crumbled feta cheese: half cup

- Lemon juice: 2 tbsp.

- Salt & black pepper, to taste

Instructions

- In a skillet, add oil (1 tbsp.) on medium flame. Add half of the chard, cook for 1-2 minutes.

- Add the rest of the chard, cook for few minutes. Add the broth.

- Cover the pan and cook for ten minutes, drain the chard in a fine sieve. Set it aside.

- Add oil (1 tbsp.) to the pan, saute garlic, and shallots. Cook for 2 minutes.

- Add drained chard, chickpeas. Cook for 3-4 minutes.

- Add lemon juice, salt, and pepper.

- Add cheese on top and serve.

Mediterranean Pork, Lamb & Beef Recipes

Burger on a Salad

(Prep time: 15 minutes | Cook time: 0 minutes |Servings: 4)

Nutrition: 305 Cal | 15 g Fat |9 g Carbs |22 g Protein

Ingredients

- English cucumber: 2 cups, chopped

- Greek dressing: half cup

- Romaine lettuce: 2 cups, chopped

- Kalamata olives: 2 tbsp., chopped

- Chopped tomatoes: 2 cups, chopped

- Red onion: half cup, chopped

- 4 beef burgers, ground & cooked

- Crumbled feta cheese: 1/4 cup

Instructions

- Microwave the burgers for 1-2 minutes until the internal temperature of the meat reaches 165 F.

- Take out and let them rest for 1 minute.

- In a bowl, add vegetables and toss with dressing (1/4 cup).

- Divide onto 4 plates, add burgers on top.

- Drizzle the remaining dressing on top.

- Top with olive and cheese, serve right away.

Herb-Crusted Pork Tenderloin

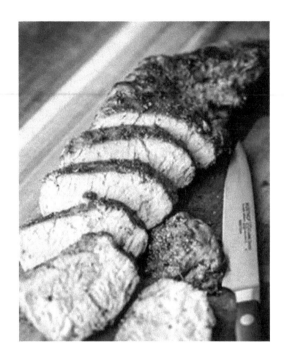

(Prep time: 15 minutes | Cook time: 20 minutes |Servings: 4)

Nutrition: 311 Cal | 11 g Fat |9 g Carbs |23 g Protein

Ingredients

- Olive oil: 1 tbsp.

- Olive tapenade: 3 tbsp.

- Dried oregano: 2 tsp.

- Pork tenderloin: 1 pound

- Lemon pepper: 3/4 tsp.

- Feta cheese: 3 tbsp., crumbled

Instructions

- Rub the pork with oil, sprinkle lemon pepper seasoning, and oregano.

- Wrap in plastic wrap and keep in the fridge for 2 hours.

- Preheat the grill to medium.

- Cut the pork in the center and make it flat.

- Spread tapenade in half, add cheese. Fold the other half over. With kitchen twine, tie the tenderloin.

- Grill for 20 minutes until the internal temperature of the meat reaches 145 F.

- Take off the grill, cover with foil, and rest for 5 to 10 minutes.

- Slice and serve.

Beef Steak & Hummus Plate

(Prep time: 15 minutes | Cook time: 0 minutes |Servings: 4)

Nutrition: 372 Cal | 18 g Fat |8 g Carbs |23 g Protein

Ingredients

- Lemon juice: 3 tbsp.

- Beef sirloin steaks: 1 pound, boneless, sliced into 1" thick

- Hummus: 1 cup

- 1 Cucumber

- Pepper: ¼ tsp.

- Romesco sauce, as needed

Rub

- Pepper: 1 tsp.

- Fresh oregano leaves: 1/4 cup, chopped

- Minced garlic: 1 tbsp. + 1 tsp.

- Grated lemon peel: 1 tbsp.

Instructions

- In a bowl, add all ingredients of rub and press into beef steak.

- Preheat the grill and grill the steak for 10-14 minutes, until the internal temperature of the meat reaches 140-160 F. Flip occasionally.

- Strip the cucumber with a peeler. In a bowl, add cucumber strips, and toss with pepper and lemon juice.

- Cut steak into thin slices, and sprinkle salt and pepper.

- On the serving plate, add ¼ cup hummus, top with beef slices, and cucumber strips. Drizzle romesco sauce on top and serve.

Mediterranean Pork With Olives

(Prep time: 10 minutes | Cook time: 20 minutes |Servings: 6)

Nutrition: 333 Cal | 13 g Fat |11 g Carbs |23.6 g Protein

Ingredients

- Olive oil: 1 tbsp.

- Ripe olives: half cup, sliced

- 6 pork chops, bone-in

- 1 onion, sliced

- Ground cinnamon, a pinch (optional)

- 2 minced garlic cloves

- 1 jar of (1 lb.) Pasta sauce

- Dry white wine: 1/4 cup

Instructions

- In a skillet, add oil on medium flame, sear the chops on all sides and take out on a plate.

- Sauté garlic and onion until tender.

- Add wine, let it come to a boil. Deglaze the pan, turn the heat low and add the pork back, pasta sauce, and the rest of the ingredients.

- Simmer for 20 minutes, covered. Serve right away with olives on top.

Mediterranean Beef Kofta

(Prep time: 20 minutes | Cook time: 20 minutes |Servings: 4)

Nutrition: 216 Cal | 12 g Fat |11 g Carbs |24 g Protein

Ingredients

- Ground beef: 1 pound

- Ground cinnamon: ¼ tsp.

- Olive oil: 1 tbsp.

- Salt: half tsp.

- Ground coriander: half tsp.

- Minced onions: half cup

- Dried mint leaves: ¼ tsp.

- Ground cumin: half tsp.

- Allspice: ¼ tsp.

Instructions

- In a bowl, add all ingredients and mix lightly but well.

- On 8" skewers, make a quarter of beef mix on the skewers. Press with fist closed to look like kofta.

- Keep in the fridge for ten minutes.

- Grill the koftas for 12-14 minutes, uncovered, until meat's internal temperature reaches 160 F.

Mediterranean Soup, Pasta & Salad Recipes

Harissa Bean Stew

(Prep time: 20 minutes | Cook time: 55 minutes |Servings: 6)

Nutrition: 202 Cal | 1 g Fat | 38 g Carbs |13 g Protein

Ingredients

Harissa

- Vegetable oil: half cup

- Ground caraway: 1 tsp.

- Smoked paprika: 2 tbsp.

- Ground coriander: 1 tbsp.

- Cayenne pepper: half-1 tsp.

- 6 minced garlic cloves

- Ground cumin: 2 tbsp.

- Kosher salt: 1 tsp.

Bean Stew

- Diced tomatoes: 1 cup, canned

- Chopped carrots: 1 cup

- Dried 15 bean mix: 1½ cups, soaked & drained

- Chopped onion: 1 cup

- Kosher salt: 1 tsp.

- Ground turmeric: 1 tsp.

- Black pepper: half tsp.

- Harissa: 1-2 tbsp. (made above)

- Apple cider vinegar: 2 tbsp.

- Chopped celery: 1 cup

- Water: 2½ cups

- Chopped fresh parsley: half cup

Instructions

- To make harissa. In a bowl, add all the ingredients, whisk well.

• Microwave for 60 seconds; after 30 seconds, stir and microwave till it is bubbly and hot.

• Let it cool completely.

• In an instant pot, add all the ingredients except for the vinegar. Mix and close the lid.

• Cook manually for half an hour on high pressure. Do the quick release after it is done cooking.

• Puree the soup with a hand mixer. Add parsley and vinegar.

• Serve right away.

Freekeh Vegetable Soup

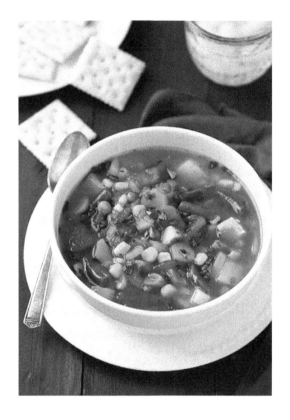

(Prep time: 10 minutes | Cook time: 45 minutes |Servings: 8)

Nutrition: 227 Cal | 9 g Fat | 28 g Carbs |11 g Protein

Ingredients

- Freekeh: 1 cup

- 1 Kohlrabi, diced

- 2 Carrots, chopped

- Kosher salt: 1 tsp.

- 2 Zucchinis, diced

- Black pepper: half tsp.

- 1 onion, chopped

- 3 Minced garlic cloves

- Olive oil: 3 tbsp.

- Cayenne pepper: ¼ tsp.

- Chicken broth: 8 cups

- Chopped fresh oregano: 2 tsp.

Instructions

- In a bowl, cover the freekeh with cold water.

- In a pot (4-5 qt.), add oil, sauté onion for 6-8 minutes. Add carrots, kohlrabi, cook for five minutes, season with salt and pepper.

- Add garlic, and cook for 60 seconds.

- Drain and wash freekeh and add in the pot.

- Add the rest of the ingredients. Let it come to a boil.

- Turn the heat low and simmer for 25-30 minutes.

- Adjust seasoning and serve right away.

Turkey Posole

(Prep time: 15 minutes | Cook time: 30 minutes |Servings: 4)

Nutrition: 227 Cal | 9 g Fat | 28 g Carbs |11 g Protein

Ingredients

- Ground turkey: 1 pound (breast)

- Chopped onion: half cup

- Green pepper: ¾ cup, chopped

- Cocoa powder: 2 tsp., unsweetened

- Poblano chile pepper: half cup, chopped

- Radishes: ¼ cup, thinly sliced

- Ground cinnamon: ¼ tsp.

- Dried oregano: 1 tsp.

- 1 Can of (~8 oz.) Tomato sauce

- Canola oil: 2 tsp.

- Salt: half tsp.

- Ground cumin: half tsp.

- 1 can of (~15 oz.) Golden hominy, rinsed

- Ground ancho chile pepper: half tsp.

- Green onions: ¼ cup, sliced

- 2 Cans of (~15 oz.) Diced tomatoes, undrained

- Chicken broth: 1 cup

Instructions

- In a Dutch oven (4 qt.), add oil, turkey, poblano, onion, and sweet pepper. Cook until meat is no longer pink.

- Drain the fat, add all spices and cook for 60 seconds.

- Add tomato sauce, tomatoes, water and hominy.

- Let it boil, turn the heat and simmer for 20 minutes.

- Serve with radishes and green onion.

Pasta alla Norma

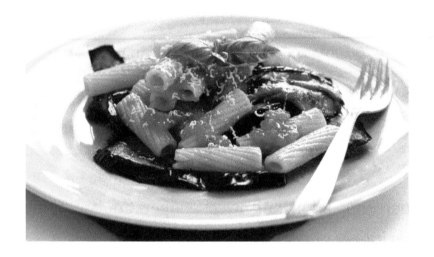

(Prep time: 10 minutes | Cook time: 30 minutes |Servings: 4)

Nutrition: 748 Cal | 21 g Fat | 22 g Carbs |26 g Protein

Ingredients

- Olive oil: 4 tbsp.

- 1 Can of (28-oz.) Crushed tomatoes

- 1 onion, sliced

- 3 Minced garlic cloves

- Salt & black pepper, to taste

- Red pepper flakes: 1 tsp.

- Dried oregano: ¾ tsp.

- Chopped fresh basil: ¼ cup

- 1 eggplant, cut into one" strips

- Grated pecorino: half cup

- Chopped fresh parsley: ¼ cup

- Small uncooked pasta: 1 pound

Instructions

- In a pan, add oil on medium flame. Add eggplant cook until golden brown.

- Take them out and season with salt and pepper.

- In the pan, sauté onion in oil for 4 minutes, add garlic and cook for 1 minute.

- Add tomatoes and let it simmer. Add the rest of the seasonings, simmer for 15-20 minutes.

- Meanwhile, cook pasta as per pack instructions.

- Add eggplant and pasts to the sauce, toss well.

- Serve with cheese on top.

Mediterranean Dessert Recipes

Brûléed Ricotta

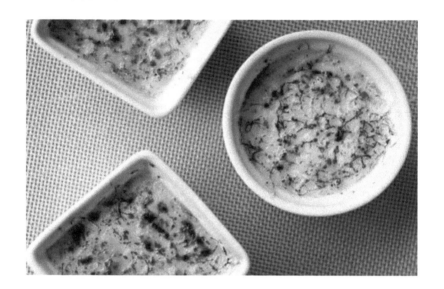

(Prep time: 5 minutes | Cook time: 10 minutes |Servings: 20)

Nutrition: 254 Cal |14.7 g Fat |23 g Carbs |12.8 g Protein

Ingredients

- Granulated sugar: 2 tbsp.

- Lemon zest: 1 tsp.

- Ricotta cheese: 2 cups

- Honey: 2 tbsp.

- Fresh raspberries, as needed

Instructions

- In a bowl, add zest, honey and ricotta mix to combine.

- Take four ramekins, and pour the batter equally. Sprinkle with sugar. Place the ramekins on the baking sheet.

- Turn on the broiler, broil the ramekins for 5-10 minutes closest to the broiler.

- Or use a kitchen torch to toast the tops.

- Cool for ten minutes, serve with fresh berries.

Egyptian Ghorayebah

(Prep time: 40 minutes | Cook time: 15 minutes |Servings: 30)

Nutrition: 82 Cal |5.6 g Fat |6.9 g Carbs |0.7 g Protein

Ingredients

- Baking powder: 1/8 tsp.

- Ghee: 1 cup

- All-purpose flour: 2 cups

- Powdered sugar: half cup

Instructions

- Whip the ghee with a hand-mixer at low speed.

- Add sugar and mix with mixer. First with low speed, then increase speed to make it fluffy and smooth.

- Add baking powder and flour (1 cup). Mix with hands and knead; add the rest of the flour. Make into a soft dough.

- Cover with plastic and keep in the fridge for 20 minutes.

- Let the oven preheat to 350 F.

- Make small balls of dough and place on a parchment-lined baking tray, flatten slightly.

- Add one almond on each cookie (if you want).

- Bake for 12-15 minutes.

- Take and let them cool before touching.

Greek Honey Sesame Bars

(Prep time: 10 minutes | Cook time: 10 minutes |Servings: 20)

Nutrition: 82 Cal |5.6 g Fat |6.9 g Carbs |0.7 g Protein

Ingredients

- Sesame seeds: 1 cup

- Greek Honey: 1 cup

- 1 lemon's zest

- Salt, a pinch

Instructions

- Toast the sesame seeds in a pan for 2 to 3 minutes until golden brown. Take them out and keep them warm.

- In the pan, add honey and let it boil till it foams. Add salt and seeds.

- Turn the heat low and mix for 3 to 5 minutes; make sure not to burn.

- Turn off the heat and add zest, mix.

- Take an 8.5" round pan and line it with parchment paper. Pour the mixture into the pan.

- Spread with a spoon, let it cool for 20 minutes.

- Cut into pieces and serve.

Mediterranean Dips, Spreads, Sauces & Snacks Recipes

Garlic Garbanzo Bean Spread

(Prep time: 10 minutes | Cook time: 0 minutes |Servings: 10-12)

Nutrition: 114 Cal | 10 g Fat |6 g Carbs |1 g Protein

Ingredients

- 1 Can of (15 oz.) Garbanzo beans, drained & rinsed

- 1 green onion, sliced into three pieces

- Fresh parsley: 2 tbsp., chopped

- Salt: 1/4 tsp.

- Olive oil: half cup

- Lemon juice: 1 tbsp.

- 1-2 garlic cloves

Instructions

- In a food blender, add all ingredients and pulse on high.

- Serve with pita bread.

Loaded Eggplant Dip

(Prep time: 15 minutes | Cook time: 20 minutes |Servings: 4-6)

Nutrition: 69 Cal | 4.7 g Fat |6.9 g Carbs |1.2 g Protein

Ingredients

- 1 Minced garlic clove

- 1 eggplant, large

- Greek yogurt: 1 ½ tbsp.

- Lemon juice: 1 tbsp.

- Salt & pepper, to taste

- Aleppo pepper: ¾ tsp.

- Tahini paste: 2 tbsp.

- Sumac: 1 tsp.

Salad Topping

- Half English Cucumber, chopped

- Fresh parsley: half cup

- Lemon juice: half tsp.

- Salt & Pepper, to taste

- 1 Tomato, chopped

- Sumac: half tsp.

Instructions

- In a bowl, add all ingredients of salad toppings, toss and drizzle olive oil.

- On low fire, toast the eggplant flip every five minutes until it is tender and the skin is charred. Turn off the heat and let it cool.

- Peel the skin off, and cut the stem. Place in a colander and drain for three minutes.

- In a food processor, add the rest of the ingredients with eggplant and pulse. Do not make a smoothie.

- Take out in a bowl, cover, and keep in the fridge for half an hour.

- Before serving, drizzle generous olive oil and add salad topping. Serve.

Asparagus with Fresh Basil Sauce

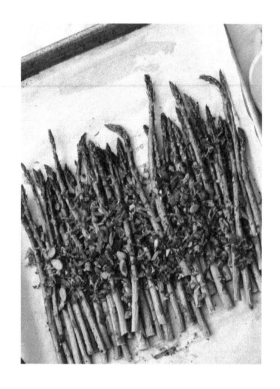

(Prep time: 5 minutes | Cook time: 2-3 minutes |Servings: 12)

Nutrition: 72 Cal | 6 g Fat |3 g Carbs |1 g Protein

Ingredients

- Reduced-fat mayonnaise: 3/4 cup

- Water: 12 cups

- Pesto: 2 tbsp.

- Fresh basil: 1 tbsp., chopped

- Fresh asparagus: 1 1/2 pounds, trimmed

- Lemon juice: 1 tsp.

- Grated parmesan cheese: 1 tbsp.

- 1 Minced garlic clove

Instructions

- In a bowl, add all ingredients except water, asparagus, mix, and keep in the fridge.

- In a pot, add water, let it boil.

- Add asparagus and cook for 2 to 3 minutes; take out and place in cold water right away.

- Dry with paper towels serve with the sauce.

Conclusion

Congratulations on finishing this book. The Mediterranean diet is quite similar to any healthy food recommendation. To follow it correctly it is necessary to follow some small precautions, such as: Consume a lot of fruit and vegetables, drink a lot of water and minimize the consumption of red meat. The Mediterranean diet is the largest but also the healthiest and most balanced that can be found. If you really want to improve your lifestyle this is the best diet for you.

Enjoy.